The Newborn: A guide to caring for your newborn

By: La'Joi Carter

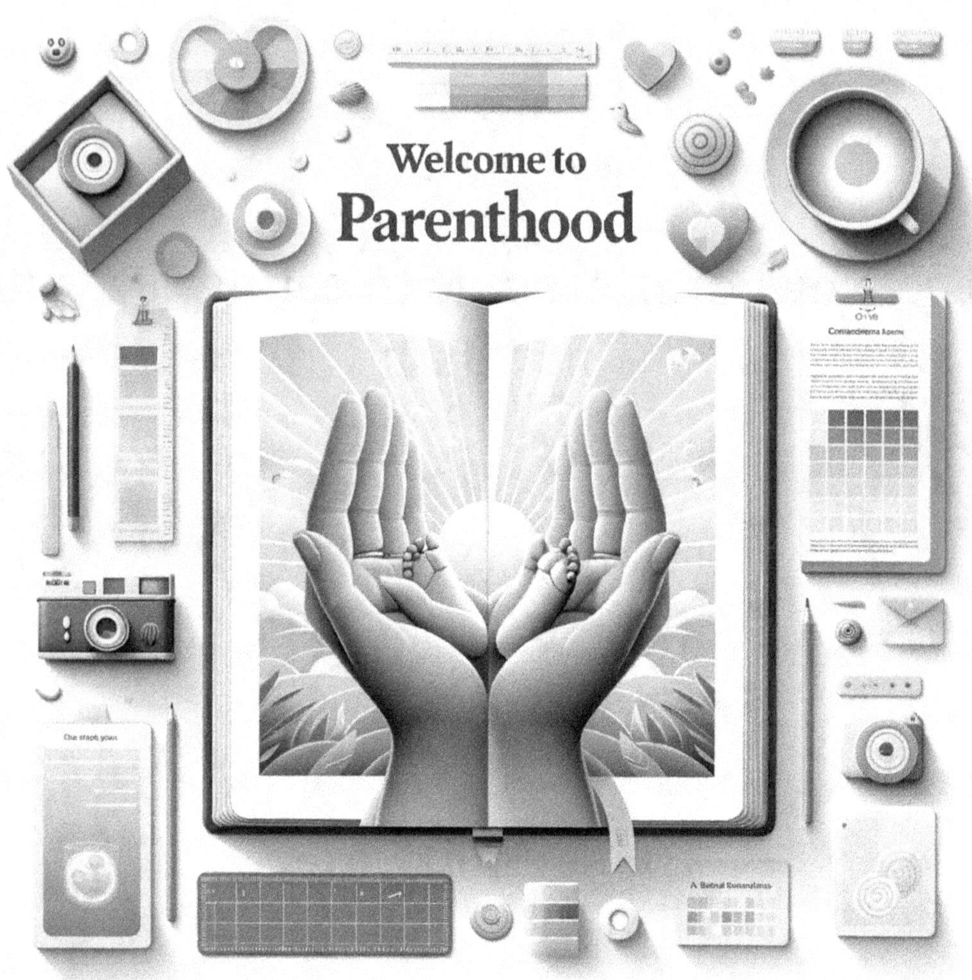

Introduction

Welcome to the journey of parenthood. Whether you're holding your newborn for the first time or preparing to welcome a new addition to your family, this book, "The Newborn: The Guidebook to Caring for a Newborn," is designed to be by your side during the incredible first year of your baby's life. Parenthood is one of the most rewarding, challenging, and transformative roles you'll ever embrace. It's a journey filled with love, surprises, and learning curves. This guidebook aims to support you every step of the way, providing practical advice, expert insights, and reassuring words to help you care for your newborn with confidence.

The first weeks and months with your newborn can feel overwhelming. You're getting to know a tiny human who depends on you for everything, while also navigating physical recovery and emotional adjustments. Our goal is to ease some of that overwhelm by equipping you with knowledge and strategies to confidently care for your newborn, understand their needs, and nurture their development.

In these pages, you'll find comprehensive information on feeding, sleeping, health, daily care routines, and developmental milestones. We've gathered wisdom from pediatricians, experienced parents, and childcare experts to offer you a trustworthy resource that answers your questions and addresses your concerns. From mastering the art of diaper changing to deciphering your baby's different cries, we're here to guide you through.

This book is also a reminder that every baby is unique, and there's no one-size-fits-all approach to parenting. We encourage you to trust your instincts, seek support when needed, and find what works best for you and your family. Alongside practical advice, we'll share stories and insights that celebrate the joys and challenges of parenting, reinforcing that you're not alone on this journey.

Remember, the days might feel long, but the years are short. Each moment with your newborn is precious and fleeting. We hope "The Newborn: The Guidebook to Help You Care for a Newborn" becomes a cherished companion, helping you navigate the early days of parenthood with love, patience, and confidence.

Welcome to the beautiful chaos of parenting. Let's begin.

Chapter 1: Understanding Newborns

Welcome to the first chapter of your journey through the early days of parenthood. Understanding your newborn is the first step towards building a strong, loving connection and providing the best care. Newborns are fascinating beings, full of surprises and equipped with their unique ways of communicating. This chapter will explore the physical and emotional characteristics of newborns, their senses, reflexes, and the vital importance of bonding during these early days.

The World Through Newborn Eyes

Newborns come into the world with a set of instincts and reflexes designed to help them navigate their new environment and bond with their caregivers. Initially, your baby's vision will be blurry, and they will see best at a distance of 8 to 12 inches— just the right distance to gaze into your eyes while feeding or being held. Over the first few months, their vision will gradually improve, allowing them to see further distances and eventually recognize faces and objects around them.

The Symphony of Newborn Sounds

Your newborn might not be able to speak, but they communicate through a symphony of sounds. From soft coos and gurgles to cries of need, every sound your baby makes is an attempt to express themselves. Learning to interpret these sounds can help you respond to your baby's needs more effectively, strengthening your bond and providing them with a sense of security and comfort.

A Touch of Comfort

Touch is a powerful tool in building a connection with your newborn. Skin-to-skin contact not only soothes and calms your baby but also promotes physiological and emotional benefits, including regulating their heart rate, temperature, and breathing. The act of holding your baby close, stroking their back, or gently massaging them can foster a deep sense of trust and attachment between you and your child.

The Reflexes of a Newborn

Newborns are born with a set of reflexes that are crucial for their survival. These include the rooting reflex, which helps them turn towards a nipple or bottle for feeding; the sucking reflex, enabling them to eat; and the startle (or Moro) reflex, a response to sudden changes in environment or position. Observing these reflexes in action can provide reassurance of your baby's neurological development and well-being.

The Bond That Binds

Bonding with your newborn is an essential part of their development and your experience as a parent. This deep, affectionate connection is the foundation for your child's emotional growth and has lasting effects on their ability to form relationships in the future. Bonding can occur in many ways—through feeding, cuddling, speaking softly to your baby, or simply spending quiet moments together. Each interaction is a building block in the lifelong relationship between you and your child.

Understanding your newborn is a journey filled with learning and discovery. As you become more attuned to your baby's needs and communication styles, you'll find your confidence growing. Remember, it's normal to feel overwhelmed at times—every parent does. Trust in your innate ability to care for and connect with your baby, and don't hesitate to seek support when needed. Your love, patience, and attentiveness are the greatest gifts you can give your newborn during these early stages of life.

Chapter 2: Feeding Your Newborn

Feeding your newborn is not just about nourishment; it's a foundational aspect of building a loving relationship and ensuring your baby's healthy development. This chapter will guide you through the essentials of feeding your newborn, covering breastfeeding, bottle feeding, understanding hunger cues, and establishing a feeding schedule.

Breastfeeding Basics

Breastfeeding is a natural process, but it's not always easy. It's a learned skill for both mother and baby, requiring patience and practice. Here, we'll discuss how to establish a good latch, which is crucial for effective breastfeeding, and explore positions that can make the experience comfortable for both you and your baby. We'll also address common challenges, such as sore nipples and low milk supply, and offer solutions to help you overcome them.

Remember, while breastfeeding is highly beneficial for both mother and baby, it's not the only option. What's most important is that your baby is fed, loved, and thriving.

Bottle Feeding Tips

Whether you're using formula or expressed breast milk, bottle feeding is an equally valid feeding method. We'll cover how to choose the right bottle and nipple to reduce gas and colic, the best techniques for holding your baby during feeds, and how to ensure your baby is getting the right amount of milk. Tips for safe formula preparation and storage will also be included to help you navigate bottle feeding confidently.

Recognizing Hunger Cues

Newborns communicate their need to eat in several ways. Early hunger cues include stirring, mouth opening, and turning their head with the mouth open, searching for a food source (rooting). Crying is a late indicator of hunger. By responding to early cues, you can feed your baby before they become too upset, which can make feeding sessions more calm and efficient.

Establishing a Feeding Schedule

Newborns typically need to be fed every 2 to 3 hours, but it's important to follow your baby's lead rather than the clock. We'll discuss the signs of a well-fed baby, how to monitor diaper output as an indicator of sufficient feeding, and when to introduce a more flexible schedule as your baby grows.

Navigating Feeding Challenges

Feeding a newborn can come with its set of challenges, from navigating growth spurts to dealing with feeding aversions. This section will offer guidance on how to adjust to your baby's changing needs and what to do if you encounter problems.

Feeding your newborn is a journey that involves learning, adjusting, and bonding. Whether breastfeeding, bottle feeding, or a combination of both, what matters most is finding a rhythm that works for you and your baby. Remember, you're not alone in this journey. Don't hesitate to seek support from lactation consultants, pediatricians, or fellow parents. With time and patience, you'll find your way, and feeding will become a cherished part of your daily routine with your newborn.

Chapter 3: Sleeping Patterns

One of the most common challenges new parents face is understanding and adapting to their newborn's sleep patterns. This chapter will delve into the basics of newborn sleep, including how to establish safe sleeping practices, interpret sleep cues, and create a conducive sleep environment. Our goal is to help you and your baby achieve more restful nights.

Understanding Newborn Sleep Cycles

Newborns sleep a lot, typically 14 to 17 hours a day, but in short bursts of 2 to 4 hours at a time. This irregular pattern is due to their small stomachs, which require frequent feedings. We'll explore the sleep-wake cycle of newborns, including the differences between REM (rapid eye movement) sleep and non-REM sleep, and why understanding these stages is crucial for your baby's development.

Safe Sleeping Practices

Sudden Infant Death Syndrome (SIDS) is a concern that weighs heavily on the minds of new parents. This section provides vital information on creating a safe sleep environment for your baby, emphasizing the importance of placing your baby on their back to sleep, using a firm sleep surface, and keeping soft objects and loose bedding out of the crib to reduce the risk of SIDS.

Soothing and Bedtime Routines

Establishing a soothing bedtime routine can signal to your baby that it's time to sleep. We'll offer tips on developing a routine that might include a warm bath, gentle massage, soft music, or reading a book. Consistency with these activities can help your baby wind down and fall asleep more easily.

Sleep Cues and How to Respond

Recognizing your baby's sleep cues is essential for preventing overtiredness. Yawning, rubbing eyes, fussiness, and staring off into space are all signs that your baby is ready for sleep. This section will guide you on how to respond to these cues to help your baby settle and sleep better.

Navigating Sleep Challenges

Many parents face sleep challenges, from difficulty settling and night waking to short naps and early rising. Here, we'll address common sleep issues and offer strategies for managing them, such as adjusting daytime naps, optimizing the sleep environment, and when it might be appropriate to gently encourage longer sleep periods at night.

While navigating your newborn's sleep patterns can be challenging, understanding the basics of newborn sleep, safe sleep practices, and the importance of a soothing routine can make a significant difference. Remember, every baby is unique, and it's okay for your approach to evolve as you learn what works best for your family. Patience, consistency, and love are key. With time, you and your baby will find a rhythm that

allows for more restful nights and joyful days.

Chapter 4: Newborn Health and Wellness

Ensuring the health and wellness of your newborn is a paramount concern for all parents. This chapter delves into common health concerns for newborns, when to seek medical advice, the importance of vaccinations, and basics of first aid for babies. Our aim is to empower you with the knowledge to care for your newborn's health confidently and to recognize when professional guidance is needed.

Common Newborn Health Concerns

Newborns can experience a variety of health issues, some more common than others. We'll explore conditions such as jaundice, diaper rash, colic, and cradle cap, providing insight into the symptoms, causes, and treatments for each. Understanding these common concerns can help you identify them early and manage them effectively, often with simple home remedies or adjustments in care.

When to Call the Doctor

Knowing when to seek medical advice is crucial for the well-being of your newborn. This section outlines clear guidelines on when to call your pediatrician, including fever, dehydration signs, difficulties in breathing, unusual lethargy, and feeding issues. We emphasize the importance of trusting your instincts as a parent; if something feels off, it's always better to err on the side of caution and consult with a healthcare professional.

The Importance of Vaccinations

Vaccinations are a key part of keeping your newborn healthy and protected against various diseases. We'll provide an overview of the recommended vaccination schedule for the first year of life, explaining the purpose of each vaccine and addressing common concerns and misconceptions about immunization. This information aims to support informed decisions about your baby's vaccination plan in consultation with your pediatrician.

Basic First Aid for Babies

Every parent should have a basic understanding of first aid for babies. This section covers essential first aid knowledge, including how to respond to choking, cuts, burns, and falls. We'll also discuss how to create a baby-safe environment to prevent accidents and the importance of having a well-stocked first aid kit tailored to the needs of a newborn.

Creating a Healthy Environment

The environment in which your baby grows plays a significant role in their overall health and development. Tips for maintaining a healthy living space include regular cleaning, minimizing exposure to allergens, and ensuring good air quality. We'll also touch on the benefits of outdoor time for your baby, including sunlight exposure for vitamin D synthesis and sensory stimulation.

Caring for your newborn's health and wellness is a comprehensive task that encompasses understanding common health issues, knowing when to seek medical advice, adhering to a vaccination schedule, and being prepared with basic first aid knowledge. By staying informed and proactive, you can ensure your baby has a healthy start to life. Remember, you're not alone in this journey; don't hesitate to reach out to healthcare professionals whenever you have concerns about your baby's

health.

Chapter 5: Daily Care Routines

Establishing daily care routines for your newborn is essential for

their health, comfort, and development. This chapter will guide

you through key aspects of daily care, including diaper

changing, bathing, dressing, and nail care, offering practical tips to make these tasks easier and more enjoyable for both you and your baby.

Diaper Changing Essentials

Diaper changing is a task you'll become very familiar with as a new parent. Here, we'll cover the basics of changing diapers, from choosing the right type for your baby to the step-by-step process of a safe and efficient diaper change. We'll also discuss common issues like diaper rash, offering advice on prevention and treatment to keep your baby comfortable.

Bath Time Basics

Bathing your newborn can be a bonding experience, but it may also seem daunting at first. This section provides a comprehensive guide to bathing your baby safely and enjoyably, including how often to bathe them, the best time for baths, and which products are safe and gentle for your baby's delicate skin. Tips for making bath time calm and enjoyable will also be included, turning it into a cherished part of your daily routine.

Dressing Your Newborn

Choosing and changing your baby's clothes might seem simple, but it comes with its own set of considerations for new parents. We'll explore how to dress your newborn for comfort and safety, considering the weather and their skin sensitivity. You'll learn how to navigate onesies, swaddles, and sleep sacks, ensuring your baby is appropriately dressed for every situation, from sleep to outdoor adventures.

Nail Care for Newborns

Newborns have soft, delicate nails that grow surprisingly fast, and keeping them trimmed is important to prevent scratching. This section will guide you on how to safely trim your baby's nails, including the best tools for the job and tips for making the process as stress-free as possible for both you and your baby.

Hair Care

While not all newborns have a full head of hair, proper scalp and hair care are important from the start. We'll discuss how to gently wash and care for your baby's hair, address common issues like cradle cap, and provide tips for brushing and maintaining healthy hair and scalp.

Mastering the daily care routines for your newborn is a significant part of parenting, fostering your baby's health, comfort, and happiness. Each task, from diaper changes to nail trimming, is an opportunity for bonding and learning. Remember, it's okay to ask for help and advice from other parents, healthcare providers, or family members as you navigate these new responsibilities. With practice and patience, you'll find a rhythm to these daily tasks, making them a natural and enjoyable part of your life with your newborn.

Chapter 6: Development and Milestones

Witnessing your newborn grow and develop is one of the most rewarding aspects of parenthood. This chapter focuses on the physical, emotional, and cognitive development milestones in the first year of life, providing you with the knowledge to support your baby's growth every step of the way.

Understanding Newborn Development

The journey begins with understanding the basic developmental stages your newborn will experience. We'll explore the rapid changes that occur in the first few months, including motor skills, sensory development, and early communication cues.

This section sets the foundation for recognizing and nurturing your baby's growth from the very start.

Physical Milestones

Physical development milestones are significant indicators of your newborn's growth. From the first reflexive movements to rolling over, sitting up, and possibly taking their first steps, we'll guide you through what to expect and when. Tips for encouraging physical development, such as tummy time and safe play, will also be discussed to help you actively support your baby's journey.

Emotional and Social Development

Emotional and social development begins with your baby's first smiles and extends to forming attachments and recognizing familiar faces. This section delves into the milestones that mark your newborn's growing emotional intelligence and capacity for social interaction. Understanding these aspects of development can enhance your bond and provide reassurance as your baby begins to explore the world around them.

Cognitive Milestones

Cognitive development in newborns involves the gradual awakening of awareness, memory, and problem-solving skills. We'll cover how your baby's brain develops in response to their environment, the importance of sensory play in fostering cognitive growth, and milestones such as recognizing cause and effect, object permanence, and the emergence of curiosity and exploration.

Language and Communication Skills

Language development starts long before your baby utters their first word. In this section, we'll examine the progression from cooing and babbling to the formation of words and simple phrases. You'll learn how to support your baby's language skills through reading, singing, and engaging in conversation, creating a rich linguistic environment that encourages communication.

Watching for Developmental Delays

While every child develops at their own pace, it's important to be aware of potential developmental delays. We'll discuss signs to watch for and how early intervention can make a significant difference. Remember, consulting with your pediatrician is crucial if you have concerns about your baby's development.

The first year of your baby's life is filled with remarkable growth and change. By understanding and supporting their development, you're providing the foundation for a healthy, happy future. Celebrate each milestone, big or small, and remember that your love and encouragement are the most powerful tools in your baby's development.

Chapter 7: Parental Health and Well-being

While much of your focus in the first year of your baby's life is on their health and development, it's crucial to also pay attention to your own well-being. This chapter addresses the importance of self-care for parents, strategies for coping with sleep deprivation, and finding support and resources. Taking care of yourself is not just beneficial for you but is essential for your ability to care for your newborn effectively.

The Importance of Self-Care

Self-care is often one of the first things to be neglected by new parents. However, maintaining your physical and mental health is crucial for both you and your baby. We'll discuss practical self-care strategies, including nutrition, exercise, and relaxation techniques, and why making time for your interests and hobbies can help you recharge and be a more present and patient parent.

Coping with Sleep Deprivation

Sleep deprivation is a common challenge in the early months of parenthood. This section offers tips for managing fatigue, such as sleeping when the baby sleeps, sharing nighttime responsibilities if possible, and creating a bedtime routine that promotes better sleep for everyone. Understanding the impact of sleep on your well-being and finding ways to maximize rest can significantly improve your quality of life during this demanding time.

Finding Support and Resources

No parent is an island, and seeking support is a sign of strength, not weakness. We'll explore various sources of support, including partners, family, friends, parenting groups, and professional services. Additionally, we'll provide guidance on how to access resources for mental health support, such as counseling or therapy, which can be invaluable for navigating postpartum depression or anxiety.

The Role of Partners in Parenting

For those with partners, this section emphasizes the importance of teamwork in parenting. Sharing responsibilities, communicating openly about each other's needs, and ensuring both partners have time for self-care are key components of a healthy parenting partnership. We'll offer tips for maintaining a strong relationship in the midst of the challenges and joys of parenting a newborn.

Single Parenting Strategies

Single parents face unique challenges and may need additional support and resources. This section is dedicated to strategies for managing the demands of solo parenting, from building a support network to finding time for self-care. We'll also highlight resources specifically aimed at assisting single parents.

Caring for a newborn is an all-encompassing task that can easily overshadow your own needs. However, your health and well-being are integral to your family's overall happiness and functioning. By prioritizing self-care, seeking support, and employing strategies to manage sleep deprivation and stress, you can navigate the challenges of new parenthood with resilience and grace. Remember, taking care of yourself is a vital part of taking care of your baby.

Chapter 8: Preparing for the Unexpected

Parenthood, especially in the early days with a newborn, is full of surprises. Despite your best efforts to prepare, unexpected situations will arise. This chapter focuses on handling emergencies, traveling with a newborn, and adjusting to life changes and challenges. Being prepared for the unexpected can help you navigate these situations with more confidence and less stress.

Handling Emergencies

The first step in handling emergencies is knowing what constitutes a medical emergency for a newborn. We'll outline the signs that indicate you should seek immediate medical attention, including but not limited to high fever, difficulty breathing, and unresponsiveness. Additionally, we'll provide tips for creating an emergency plan, including having a list of emergency contacts, knowing the location of the nearest pediatric emergency room, and taking a course in infant CPR and first aid.

Traveling with a Newborn

Traveling with a newborn presents a unique set of challenges and requires careful planning. This section covers everything from packing essentials and choosing baby-friendly accommodations to tips for feeding and soothing your baby on the go. We'll also discuss safety considerations for car travel and flying with a newborn, helping you to plan a trip that's safe and comfortable for everyone involved.

Adjusting to Life Changes and Challenges

The arrival of a newborn can bring significant life changes, affecting your relationships, career, and personal identity. We'll explore strategies for navigating these changes, such as communicating openly with your partner, setting realistic expectations for yourself, and finding a balance between parenting responsibilities and personal time. Recognizing and accepting that adjustments are part of the journey can make the transition into parenthood smoother.

Building Flexibility and Resilience

Flexibility and resilience are key qualities for new parents. This section offers advice on how to cultivate these traits, emphasizing the importance of being adaptable in the face of unexpected challenges and maintaining a positive outlook.

Learning to let go of perfection and embrace the unpredictability of parenthood can lead to a more enjoyable and less stressful experience.

Preparing for the unexpected is an essential part of parenthood. While it's impossible to anticipate every situation, being informed, creating a support network, and developing flexibility can help you navigate the unforeseen challenges that arise. Remember, it's okay to ask for help, and taking things one step at a time can make even the most daunting situations manageable. Parenthood is a journey of constant learning and growth, and every challenge is an opportunity to strengthen your resilience and deepen your bond with your newborn.

Chapter 9: Conclusion

As we wrap up "The Newborn: The Guidebook to Help You Care for a Newborn," it's important to reflect on the journey we've embarked upon together. From understanding newborns to preparing for the unexpected, each chapter has been crafted to equip you with the knowledge, skills, and confidence needed to navigate the early days of parenthood. This concluding chapter aims to recap key points, offer encouraging final thoughts, and provide additional resources to support you as you continue this remarkable journey.

Recap of Key Points

Throughout this guidebook, we've covered a broad range of topics essential to newborn care, including:

- Understanding your newborn's physical and emotional needs.

- The basics of feeding, whether breastfeeding or bottle-feeding, and recognizing hunger cues.

- Navigating sleep patterns and establishing safe sleeping practices.

- Addressing common health concerns and when to seek medical advice.

- Daily care routines that foster your newborn's well-being.

- Monitoring development and milestones to support your baby's growth.

- Prioritizing your health and well-being as a parent.

- Preparing for unexpected situations and building resilience.

Each chapter has been designed to support you through the various aspects of caring for a newborn, offering practical advice and reassuring guidance.

Encouraging Final Thoughts

Parenthood is a journey filled with love, challenges, and incredible rewards. It's normal to feel overwhelmed at times, but remember, you are not alone. Trust in your instincts, lean on your support network, and don't hesitate to seek professional advice when needed. Celebrate the small victories, cherish the moments of connection, and know that every day you are doing your best for your child.

As your baby grows and changes, so too will your experience of parenthood. Embrace the journey, with all its ups and downs, for it is truly one of life's most profound and enriching experiences.

Resources

To further support you on your parenting journey, here are some additional resources:

- **Pediatric Health Organizations:** Websites like the American Academy of Pediatrics (AAP) offer a wealth of information on child health, development, and safety guidelines.
- **Parenting Forums and Support Groups:** Online communities can be a great source of support, advice, and camaraderie with other parents navigating similar challenges.
- **Local Parenting Classes:** Many hospitals and community centers offer classes on infant care, CPR, and parenting skills.
- **Books and Podcasts:** There are numerous books and podcasts dedicated to early parenthood that can provide insights, advice, and comfort.

Remember, this guidebook is a starting point. Continue to seek out information, ask questions, and find what works best for you and your family.

Thank you for allowing "The Newborn: The Guidebook to Help You Care for a Newborn" to be a part of your parenting journey. It's been an honor to provide you with guidance during this special time in your life. May the days ahead be filled with joy, love, and the wonderful adventure of raising your newborn. Here's to the journey ahead—may it be everything you hope for and more.

For new parents seeking additional resources and considering hiring a doula for extra support in caring for their newborn, here's a comprehensive list to help guide your journey:

Additional Resources for Newborn Care

1. **American Academy of Pediatrics (AAP) - HealthyChildren.org:** Offers up-to-date information on child health, developmental milestones, and safety guidelines.

2. **La Leche League International:** A valuable resource for breastfeeding support, including finding local groups and accessing expert advice.

3. **Centers for Disease Control and Prevention (CDC) - Infant and Toddler Nutrition:** Provides guidelines on feeding, nutrition, and introducing solid foods.

4. **Zero to Three:** Focuses on early development and well-being, offering resources on infant mental health and developmental stages.

5. **BabyCenter:** Features articles, tools, and forums on various aspects of pregnancy, newborn care, and parenting.

6. **Local Parenting Classes:** Many hospitals, community centers, and childcare organizations offer classes on newborn care, CPR, and parenting skills.

Finding and Hiring a Doula

Doulas provide emotional, physical, and educational support to families before, during, and after childbirth. While they do not offer medical care, their support can be invaluable in helping parents adjust to life with a newborn.

1. **DONA International:** One of the oldest and largest doula associations offering a directory to find certified birth and postpartum doulas.

2. **Childbirth and Postpartum Professional Association (CAPPA):** Offers education and certification for childbirth educators, doulas, and lactation educators. Their website includes a directory to find professionals in your area.

3. **DoulaMatch.net:** A free service that matches you with both birth and postpartum doulas based on your due date and location.

4. **Local Doula Networks:** Many regions have local doula networks or collectives, which can be found through online searches or recommendations from healthcare providers or parenting groups.

Tips for Hiring a Doula

- **Interview Several Doulas:** Meet with a few doulas to find someone with whom you feel comfortable and whose experience aligns with your needs.

- **Check References:** Ask for and follow up with references to hear about other families' experiences.

- **Discuss Services and Fees:** Clearly understand what services they offer, their availability, and how their fees are structured.

- **Consider Compatibility:** Since you'll be sharing intimate experiences, choose a doula with whom you feel a strong sense of trust and comfort.

Online Forums and Support Groups

- **Mothering Forums:** Offers a community for parents to discuss various topics, including newborn care, breastfeeding, and the role of doulas.

- **Reddit Parenting Communities:** Subreddits like r/Parenting, r/NewParents, and r/BabyBumps can be valuable for advice and support from a broad community of parents.

By leveraging these resources and considering the support of a doula, you can enrich your knowledge, build your confidence, and enhance your support network as you navigate the early days of parenthood.